BIG WIG

A LITTLE HISTORY OF HAIR

BY KATHLEEN KRULL

ILLUSTRATED BY PETER MALONE

ARTHUR A. LEVINE BOOKS   AN IMPRINT OF SCHOLASTIC INC.

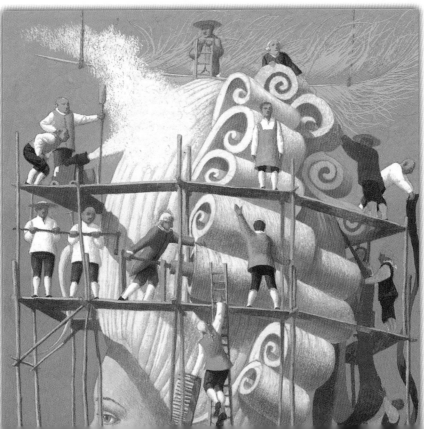

To poodley Pablo —KK
To my barber, S. Todd —PM

The publisher gratefully acknowledges Victoria Sherrow for her expert advice on the history of hair and hairstyles.

Text copyright © 2011 by Kathleen Krull
Illustrations copyright © 2011 by Peter Malone

LIBRARY OF CONGRESS CATALOGING-IN-PUBLICATION DATA

Krull, Kathleen.
Big wig : a little history of hair / by Kathleen Krull ; illustrated by Peter Malone. — 1st ed.   p.   cm.
Includes bibliographical references and index.
ISBN 978-0-439-67640-3 (hardcover : alk. paper)
1. Hair—History—Anecdotes. I. Malone, Peter, 1953- II. Title.
GT2290.K78 2011   391.5—dc22   2010031005

10 9 8 7 6 5 4 3 2 1   11 12 13 14 15

Printed in Singapore 46
First edition, August 2011

The text type was set in 13-point Adobe Garamond Pro Regular and Semibold.
The display type was set in Eccentric Std.
The art for this book was created using gouache.

Book design by Marijka Kostiw

NOTE FROM THE AUTHOR

At age ten, I made my first "book," called *Hair-Dos and People I Know*, a collection of girl and boy

hairdos, nun hairdos, and tree hairdos. I have since come to find out that lots of others are interested

in hair. Hair is a big clue about our identity—it's really the only part of ourselves we have some control

over, and the possibilities for variety are endless. Careful readers will notice frequent mentions of hair

in my books, as in my fictional *Clip Clip Clip*. As for researching hairstyles throughout the ages,

I've been "clipping" articles about this for years—I'm grateful to Arthur Levine and his colleagues

at Scholastic for suggesting this book. Also Caitlin Krull, Robert Pinsky, Kathy Hewitt, and others

who have sent hairy tips over the years. The wide range of other sources for the facts here are listed at

the back of the book. And now I invite you to enjoy—and see if you agree with me that the history

of the world is the history of hair.

PREHISTORY,
AFRICA

In the beginning, everyone is furry. People make friends by grooming each other. That is, picking the bugs out of another guy's fur coat.

Fur coats are just so buggy and hot. Over time, they grow smaller and smaller, until they're mainly on top, for sun protection. Now it's easier to make friends, even with terrible bed head.

Men and women gather plants to eat. Except those who draw on the walls of their caves instead. One day, cave painters notice that their paintbrushes aren't bad at grooming hair. They invent the first hairbrush.

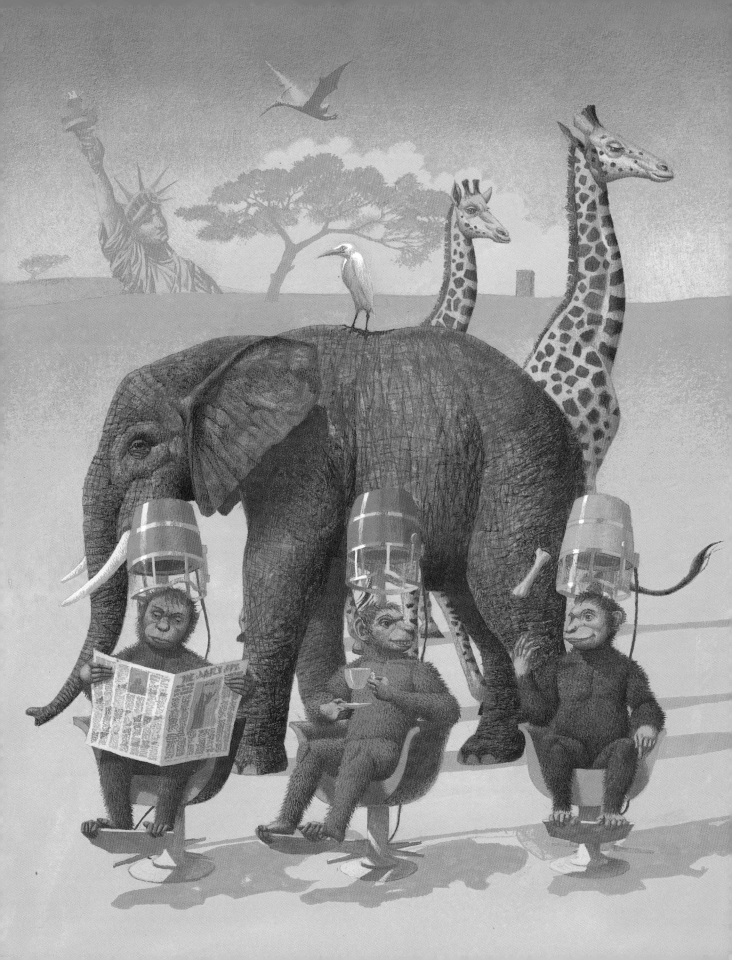

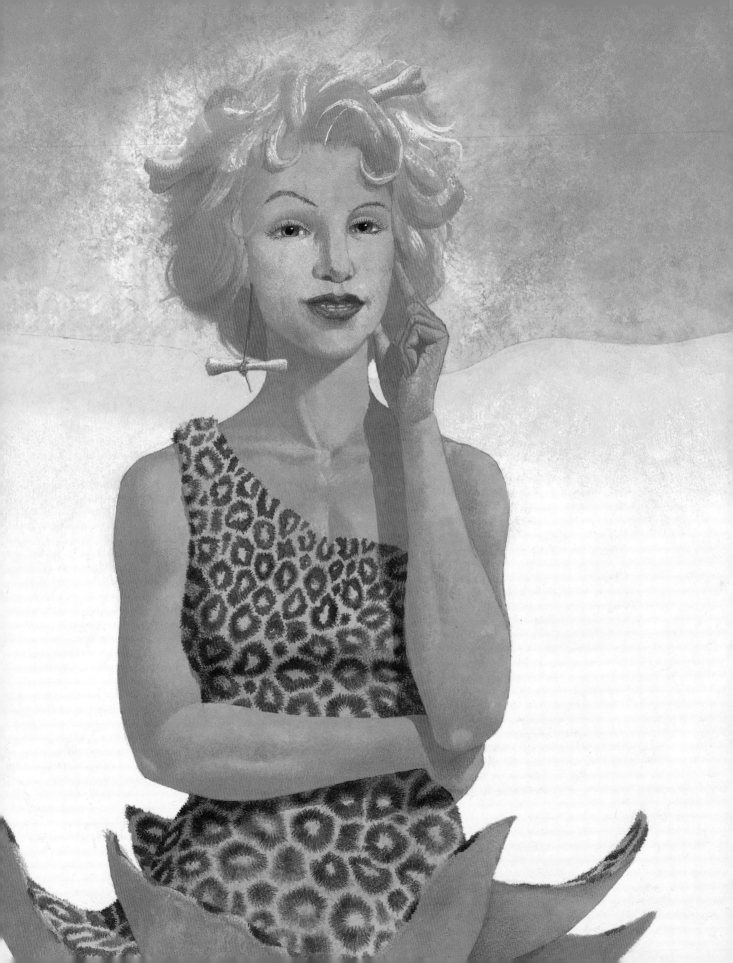

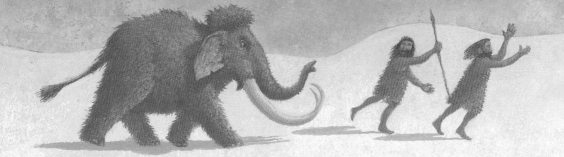

11,000 YEARS AGO,
SOMEWHERE IN NORTHERN EUROPE

For millions of years, as humans move from Africa to other places, everyone's hair stays one color: dark brown.

Then a cavewoman sprouts yellow hair. Why? The men have started to hunt for meat. The dangers of going after reindeer, mammoths, and horses are killing too many cavemen. Cavewomen have to compete for the few men left. Instead of beating each other up, they evolve ways to be more special. Being blond seems to help.

ABOUT 5,000 YEARS AGO, PRESENT-DAY NIGERIA

The Yoruba-speaking people think of hairstyles as an art form. Children born with knotted hair are considered lucky and allowed to keep their hair uncut, forming dreadlocks. Some women arrange their braids in complex patterns, later to be known as cornrows.

5,000 YEARS AGO, EGYPT

Egyptians shave their heads. Good-bye, bugs. But how to protect bald heads from the hot sun? Wigs, stiffened with beeswax—brilliant! Wigmakers use real hair taken from slaves or dead people, or sheep's wool, or palm leaves. The most popular colors are black and red—from dried henna leaves mixed with cow's blood. Later, bright green and blue wigs become trendy. Those who can afford it sprinkle their wigs with real gold dust. Kings wear fake beards—and so do queens.

4,000 YEARS AGO,
PRESENT-DAY MEXICO AND CENTRAL AMERICA

The Mayan look is unique—buttery-soft hair atop a long skull. Your mom sandwiches your head between boards—for days. When your head is long enough, she rubs an avocado in your hair to keep it velvety. Then she ties a bead in the hair hanging over your eyes. So they will cross—part of the look.

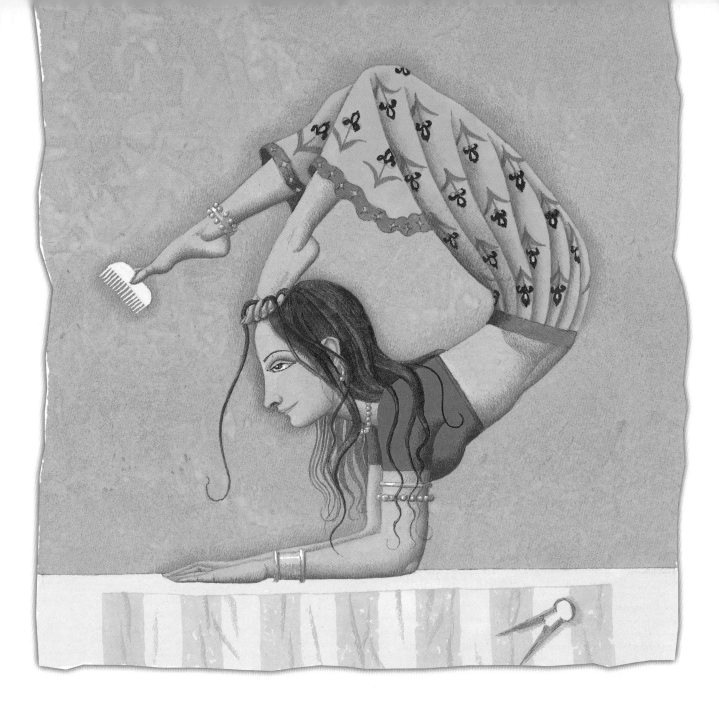

4,000 YEARS AGO, INDIA

Everyone in the world wants to brush and decorate their hair with fancy combs made here. People don't use chemicals or dyes, but do use massage and headstands to make hair healthier. In a Hindu ceremony, the hair of all children is shaved off before age seven. Hair from India becomes the main source for wigs everywhere else.

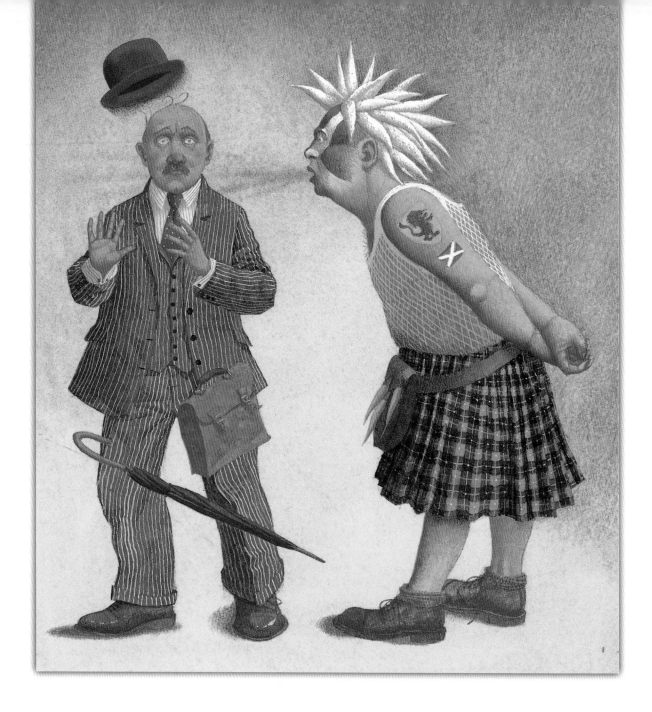

3,000 YEARS AGO,
PRESENT-DAY IRELAND AND SCOTLAND

The Celts want to do a better job of scaring their enemies. So they apply chalk to their long hair to whiten it, then they shape it into stiff spikes. For maximum terror, they also paint scary blue designs on their faces and shout, "Boo!"

2,400 YEARS AGO, GREECE

Rubbing goat pee on his head. That's how the wise philosopher Aristotle thinks he will cure his baldness. But Hippocrates, known as the Father of Medicine, prefers his own brews, which include opium, wine, green olive oil, horseradish, and pigeon poop.

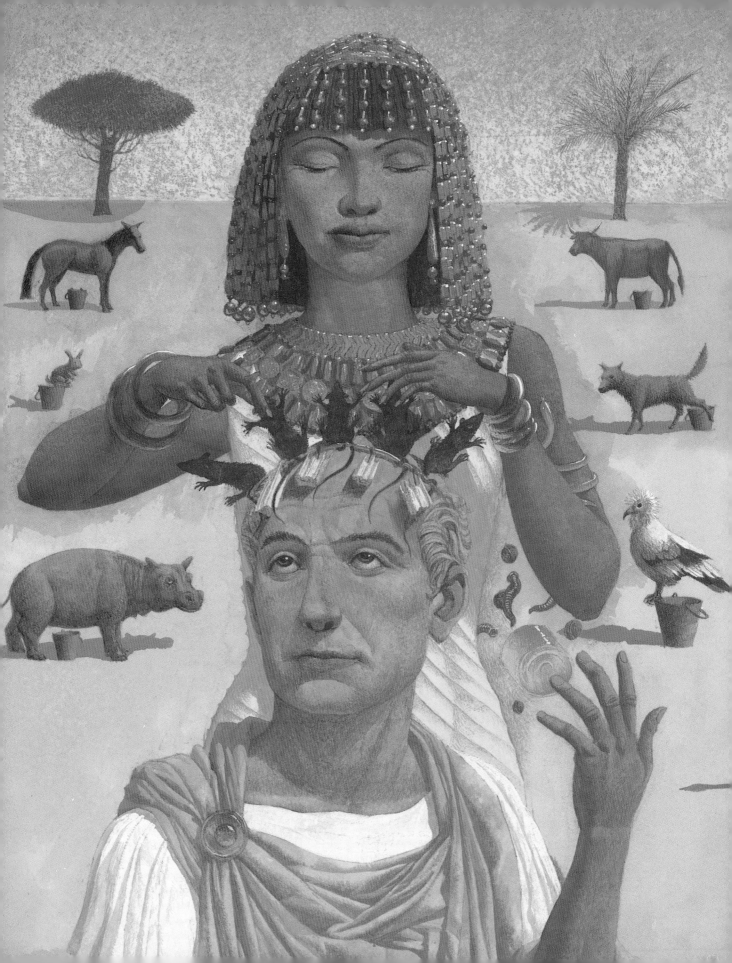

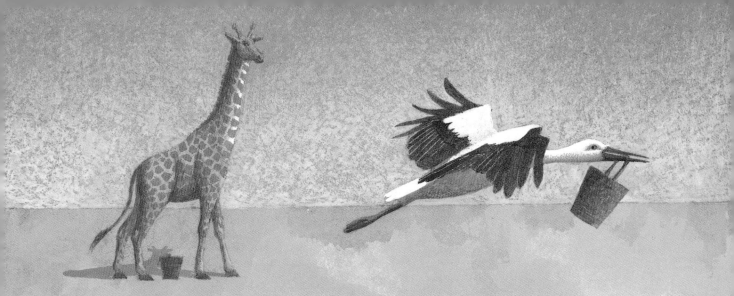

ABOUT 2,000 YEARS AGO, ROME

Queen Cleopatra drops hints to her boyfriend, Julius Caesar. Wouldn't the emperor of Rome like to cure his baldness with a blend of horse teeth and deer marrow, all spiced up with toasted mice? He would. He stops using his old method—a paste made from leeches, boiled walnut shells, tar, and pee from various animals.

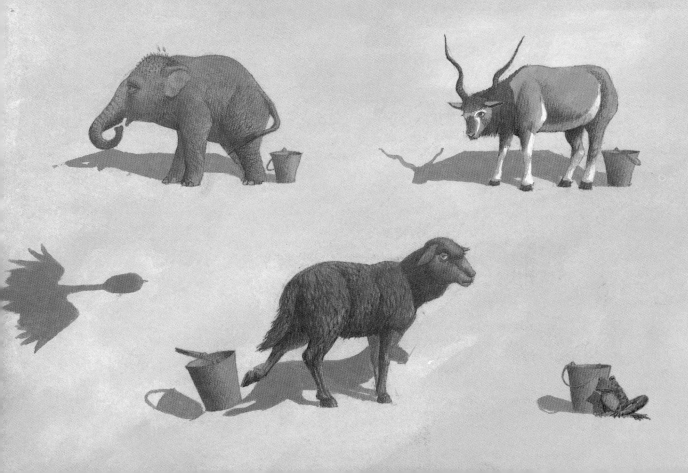

1200s to 1800s, Japan

Every samurai warrior begins his morning the same way: shaving the top of his head, smearing oil on the remaining hair, and tying it into a special topknot, locked into place with long hairpins. No one else *dares* to look like a samurai.

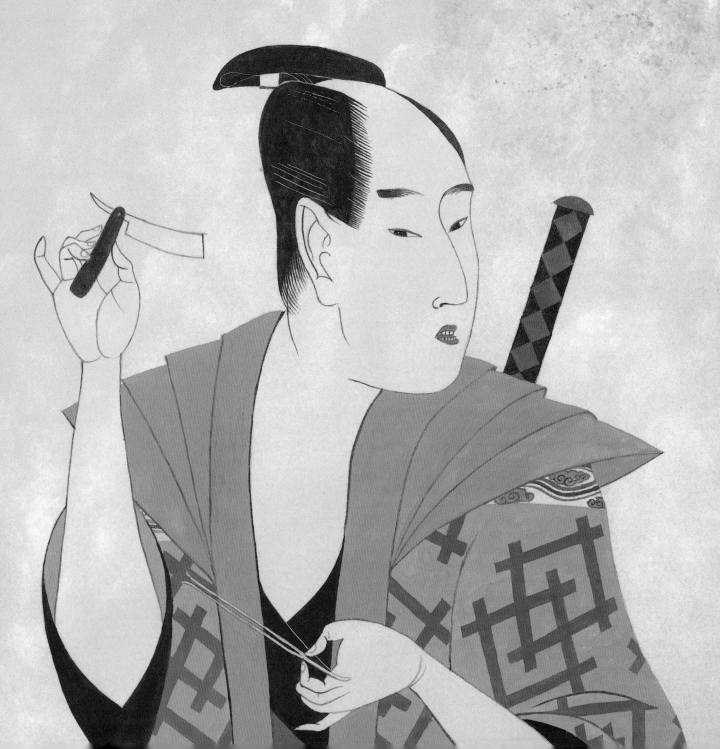

1428, France

Most people are shocked when Joan of Arc chops off her long hair. Women are *not* supposed to look like men. Joan doesn't care—she has run away from home and is on her way to leading the French army to victory.

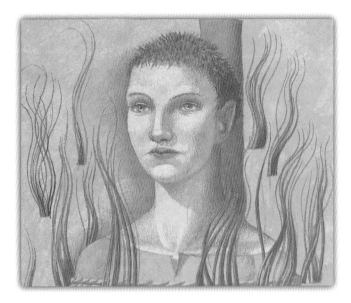

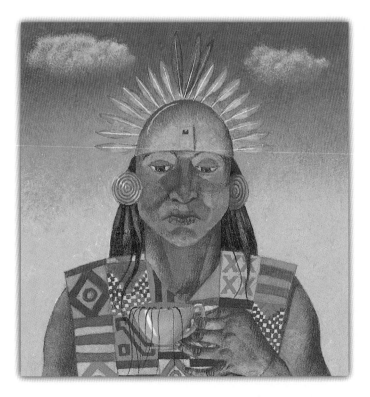

1438, present-day Peru, South America

For the next hundred years, during the height of the Inca Empire, hair is used in medicine. The victim of a poisoning, for example, is fed fermented corn mixed with ashes from the burning of a lock of his or her hair.

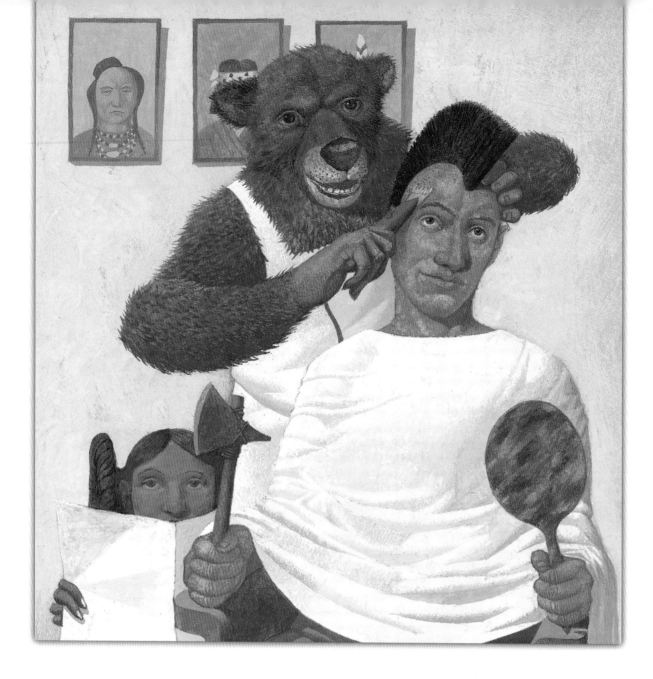

Before 1500, present-day United States

American Indians use bear grease, mixed with sweet-smelling leaves like mint, as the best conditioner, as well as a bug-killer. Many tribes set themselves apart with cool hairstyles. The Mohawk, of present-day New York State, shave their heads, leaving one ridge of hair sticking up. Young Hopi girls, of present-day New Mexico, wear two large whirls on either side of the head, like squash blossoms.

1500s, VENICE, ITALY

Trendy Renaissance women dye their hair with precious saffron flowers mixed with lye, a harsh chemical. Then they sit in the boiling sun all day, wearing special hats that expose the hair. While sweat pours off them, they admire their blondness in mirrors.

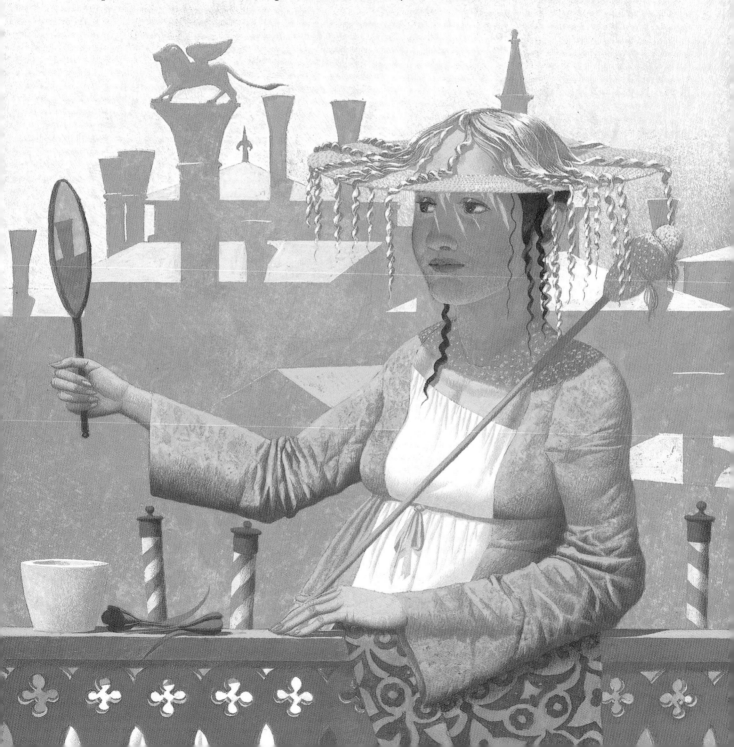

1558, ENGLAND

Since mighty Queen Elizabeth is a redhead, red hair rules. Men in her court hurry to dye their beards red to show loyalty. As her hair thins, she gets more than eighty wigs in various shades of red—and dyes the tails of her horses to match.

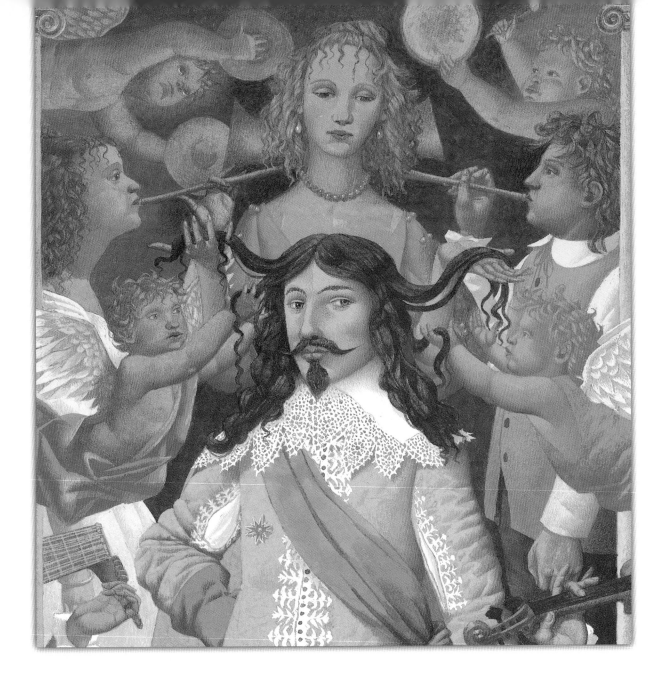

1624, France

King Louis XIII starts losing his long curls when he's only 23. Obsessed with his image (and related to King Charles the Bald), he throws on a big wig. Everyone at court jumps to copy him, even men with great hair. Made from human hair or wool, wigs are heavy, uncomfortable, and kind of embarrassing. But soon the wealthy in England copy the French. Flowing wigs are back in a big way, even for children.

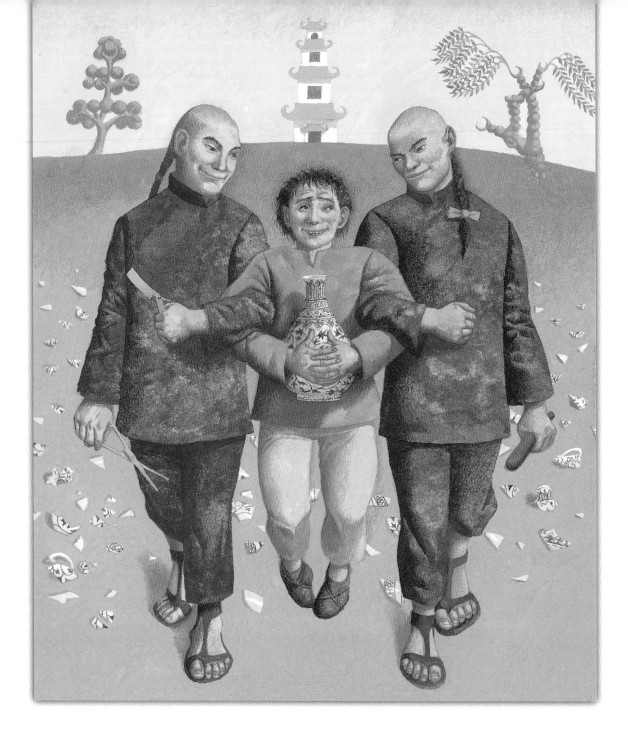

1644, CHINA

The new Manchu government orders *all* men to shave the top of their heads and grow a long pigtail in back. By force, if necessary. It's the way to show you are no longer loyal to the previous dynasty, the Ming.

About 1785, Versailles, France

Do Queen Marie Antoinette and women at court have too much time on their hands? They coax their hair over a "rat"—a wire form rising several feet, padded with cloth or horsehair, held together with lard, dusted with potato flour. Then they glue things inside—miniature rooms of furniture, a vegetable garden, or the planets revolving. How about a birdcage with live birds, or the model of a ship? Or barnyards, children's toys, famous battles? The hairdos stay in place for months: Imagine the itchiness.

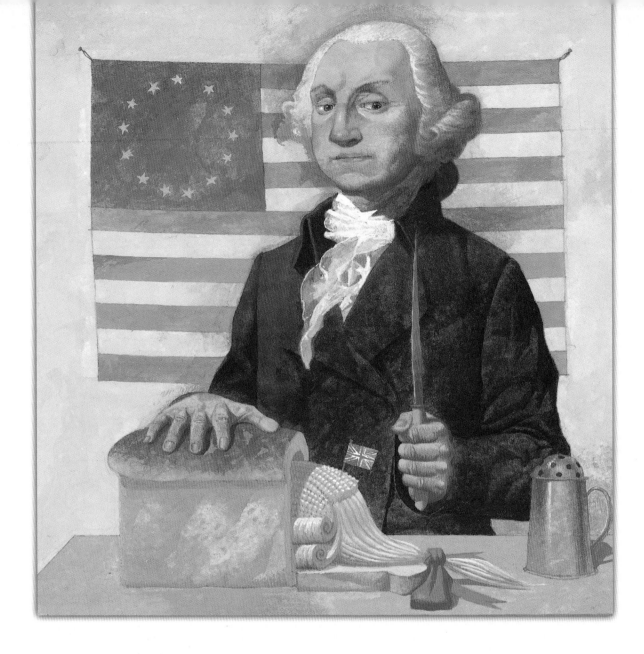

1789, United States

Over in the colonies, wigs remind patriots of the hated British. But it's still not cool to show your natural hair. The new president powders his brown hair white and ties it back in a little black bag. No wig for George Washington. Some pompous men cling to their giant wigs. They debate how best to clean them, like baking them inside a loaf of bread that has been hollowed out—the heat makes the wig hairs expand even more. "Big wig" becomes the term for a pompous person.

AROUND 1810, VIENNA, AUSTRIA

Many artists and musicians think wigs are stupid. One is the classical composer LudWIG van Beethoven, with his long, wild hair. So many musicians wear the unfashionable longer style that for years classical music is known as "longhaired music."

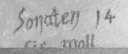

1814, BRIGHTON, ENGLAND

Shampoo—so far a crude brew—improves as people get access to running water. Sake Dean Mahomed opens "The Indian Medicated Vapour Bath," where customers can pay to get hair washed. He is appointed "shampooing surgeon" to two English kings.

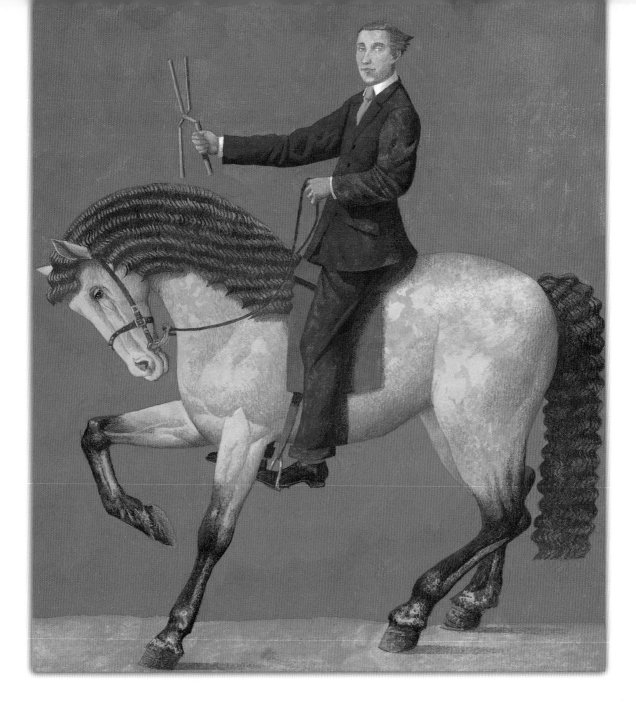

1872, Paris, France

Marcel Grateau's job is grooming horses. At age 20, he switches to grooming his mom. One day, he accidentally creates an effect in her hair that looks like real waves. He goes on to invent a type of curling iron that heats over a gas burner. His customers adore what they call the "Marcel wave" and make it all the rage for the next 50 years.

1882, LOCKPORT, NEW YORK

The seven singing Sutherland sisters join the circus. Their dad notices that something gets more applause than their singing—their hair, said to be the longest in the world. He invents "Seven Sutherland Sisters Hair Grower" as a cure for baldness. Does it work? No matter. With the profits, Sarah, Victoria, Isabella, Grace, Naomi, Dora, and Mary end up living in a fabulous mansion.

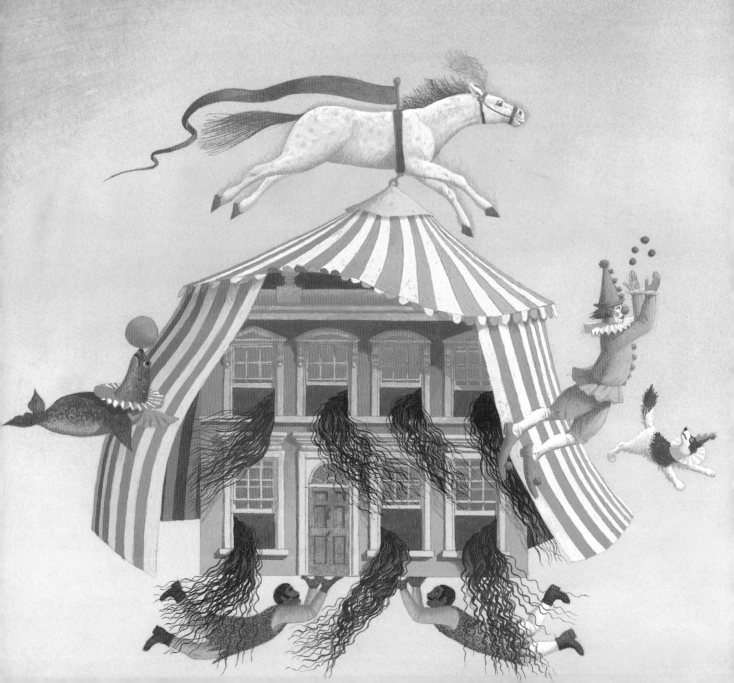

1905, DENVER, COLORADO

Sarah Breedlove washes other people's clothes, as usual, and frets about her thinning hair, as usual. One night, she has a dream about a recipe that will make it look much better. The next morning, she makes a conditioning potion. She starts selling it by going from one house to the next. Twelve years from now, as Madam C. J. Walker, she will be one of the first African-American millionaires in history.

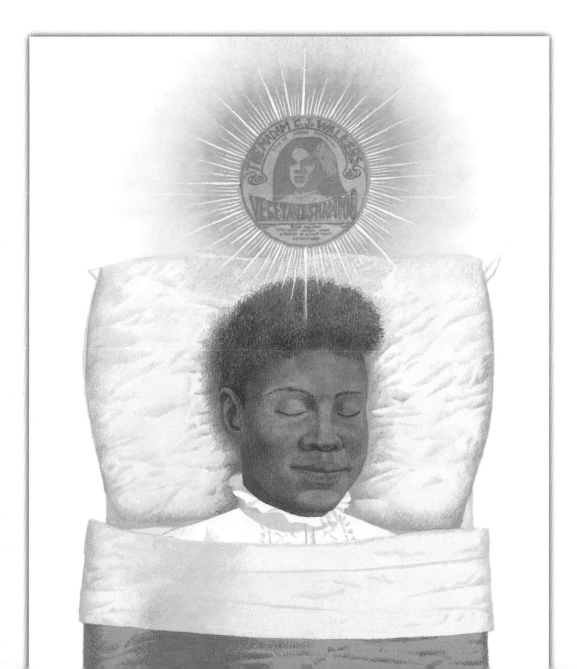

AROUND 1935, MEXICO

For Frida Kahlo, the painter, hair is yet another art form. Every day, she tweaks it differently, often in styles from different areas of Mexico, pulling it back hard enough to hurt a lot. She spends hours and hours adorning it with fresh flowers, jewels, and bows.

1936, HOLLYWOOD, CALIFORNIA

Each night, Mrs. Temple rolls her eight-year-old daughter's hair into tight pin curls. Exactly 56 curls in all. The girl wakes up with flawless ringlets. She is Shirley Temple, and for the next three years she is the top-earning movie star in the world.

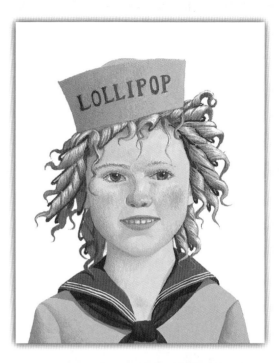

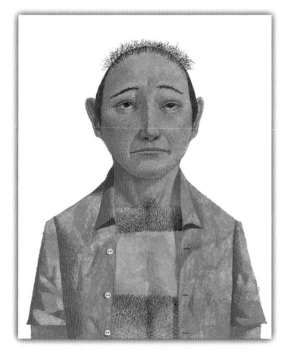

1939, JAPAN

People are more frantic than ever to cure baldness. Finally, Japanese skin doctors invent a way to implant live hairs from one part of the body to another—the first modern hair transplants. Then World War II interrupts. No one in the rest of the world learns about the Japanese breakthrough until 1945, when the war ends.

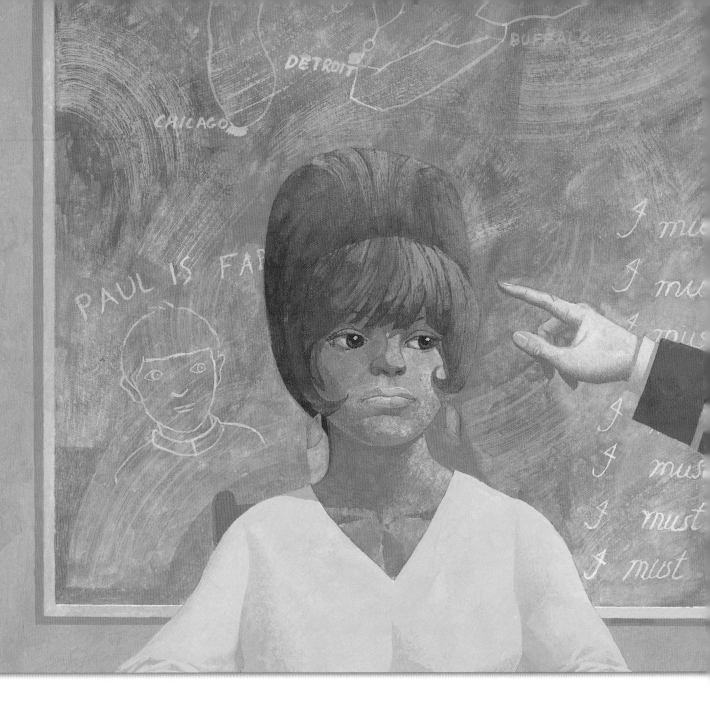

1961, DETROIT, MICHIGAN

The Supremes are born, sporting big hair swept up into a pouf. Girls across America
aim high for bouffants or beehives, using giant hair rollers, harmful backcombing
(or teasing), and fantastic amounts of hairspray. Some schools ban beehives because
they prevent other students from seeing the blackboard.

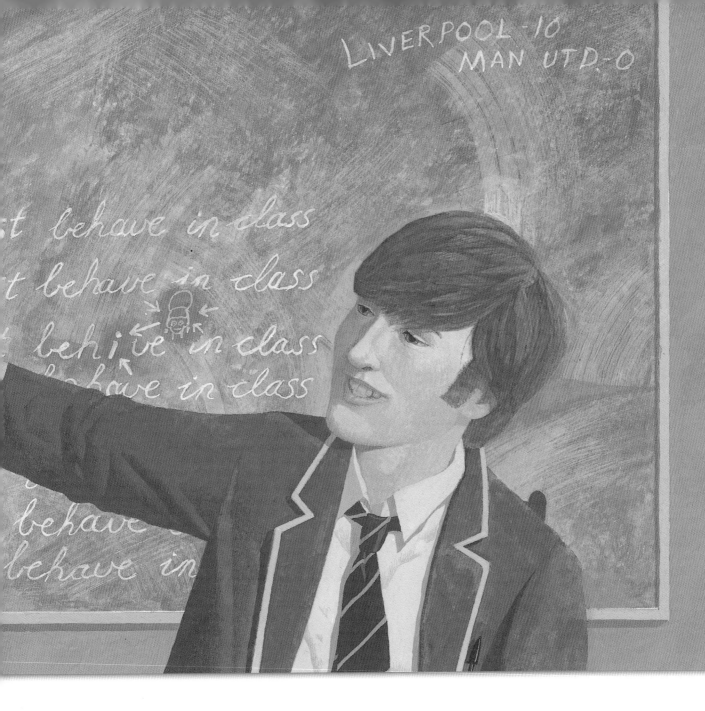

1964, LIVERPOOL, ENGLAND

Four cute young men fly to New York to appear on American TV for the first time. The Beatles change everything. Yes, their music rocks, but at first, it's their moptop hair that makes girls scream.

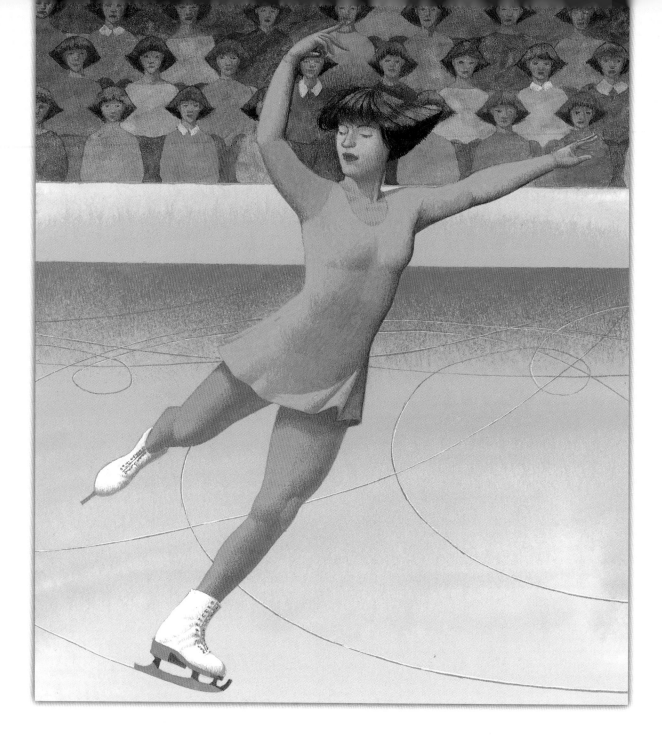

1974, GREENWICH, CONNECTICUT

Eighteen-year-old Dorothy Hamill asks her hairdresser to *please* keep the hair out of her eyes. She goes on to win the Olympic gold medal for figure skating. As she whirls, her wedge cut inspires girls everywhere, especially athletes.

1970s AND '80s, NEW YORK CITY AND LONDON

Hair is serious to the punk look, which aims to shock. Too cool for words, rebels use Kool-Aid powder to achieve colors not found in nature. To get their spiky variations on the Mohawk, they use egg whites or a mixture of water plus sugar, flour, or soap.

2007, ENGLAND

Someone gets the most expensive haircut ever—$16,300.00. Luckily, the price includes lunch.

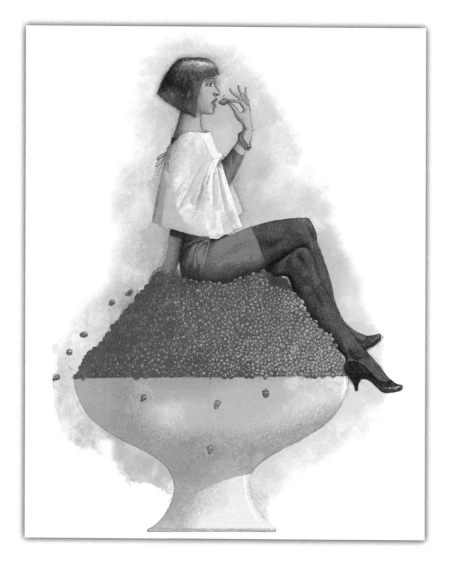

NOW IT'S YOUR TURN.

HOW WILL YOU MAKE HISTORY WITH YOUR HAIR?

BIG WIG

HAIR EXTENSIONS

AFRICA, IN THE BEGINNING In parts of ancient Africa, the very definition of "human being" was "one whose hair grows mainly on the head."

11,000 YEARS AGO, SOMEWHERE IN NORTHERN EUROPE Naturally blond hair has been found all over the world, including in Africa and among the aboriginal people of Australia. But it remains most common in the countries of northern Europe.

ABOUT 5,000 YEARS AGO, PRESENT-DAY NIGERIA Because hair was believed to contain a person's spirit, hairdressers were some of the most important people in a village. Artistic children were encouraged to go into hairdressing—creating even more styles.

5,000 YEARS AGO, EGYPT At the wilder parties, Egyptians would place atop their wigs a cone of fat mixed with cinnamon chips. As the party went on, the cone melted and sweetened the air.

4,000 YEARS AGO, PRESENT-DAY MEXICO AND CENTRAL AMERICA You could tell a Mayan noble by the complexity of hairstyle and the size of his elaborate feather headdress—if it was as tall as he was, this was someone you didn't mess with.

4,000 YEARS AGO, INDIA India later became *the* source for healthy hair, with 450 tons sold in 2003. Even today, thousands of pilgrims line up at temples for the Hindu custom of sacrificing their hair. One of its main destinations is Hollywood.

3,000 YEARS AGO, PRESENT-DAY IRELAND AND SCOTLAND Later, pirates may have used hair as a weapon like the Celts did. In the early 1700s, the English pirate known as Blackbeard scared colonial Americans silly by tying colored ribbons to locks of his thick black hair, inserting lit matches, and roaring as he attacked their ships.

2,400 YEARS AGO, GREECE The wise historian Plutarch recommended washing hair only once a year, so as not to disturb the spirit that guarded the head. For men in ancient Greece, haircuts were a big social event, for exchanges of news and gossip, philosophy, and hair tips. (Women had their hair groomed at home by servants.)

ABOUT 2,000 YEARS AGO, ROME The queen of Egypt was also queen of fabulous hair, with so much to say about it that she wrote a whole book of beauty tips.

ABOUT 500 TO 1300, EUROPE About the only interesting development in the Middle Ages was when some wealthy people tied gold balls to the ends of their hair. Remedies for hair ailments continued to use poop (from swallows and cats), as well as lizards boiled in oil, and lanolin—the grease that floats to the top when boiling sheep's wool. Even the wealthy rarely bathed, but those who did considered Spain to have the best soap, made with olive oil.

AROUND 800, PRESENT-DAY IRAQ Unlike in most other areas of the world, regular bathing has been common in Arab countries since ancient times. Men and women had their hair washed in hammams, or public baths. Eventually, Europeans who came here to fight in the Crusades took this bath idea back with them when they went home. Even by 1451, when Queen Isabella of Spain was born, the concept hadn't quite caught on—she was rumored to have taken only two baths during her life.

1200S TO 1800S, JAPAN Later, presumably when samurai warriors were less intimidating, many men in Japan adopted their hairstyle. Meanwhile, Japanese women, who did not typically wear jewelry on their bodies, wore works of art in their hair instead—gorgeous, intricate ornaments.

1428, FRANCE Also in France, almost a hundred years later (1521), the hair of King Francis I was accidentally set on fire. It happened one wild night during a snowball fight, when someone carelessly threw a flaming torch. The next day, all men in court cut their hair short in sympathy with the king.

1438, PRESENT-DAY PERU, SOUTH AMERICA The Inca placed great significance on hair. In a ceremony held for two-year-old babies, relatives took turns cutting off locks of the child's hair. After they put them away in a safe place, the oldest uncle would cut his own hair and sacrifice it to the gods to ask for the baby's good health.

BEFORE 1500, PRESENT-DAY UNITED STATES After 1865, when a new law required American Indian children to attend government-run schools, they were forced to cut their hair in the style of white Americans in an attempt to erase their cultural identity.

1500S, VENICE, ITALY The mania for blond reversed a trend from the earlier days of the Roman Empire, when blond hair was viewed negatively—women of ill repute were *required* to have it. But as Rome began acquiring women slaves from northern Europe—such as the Scandinavian countries or Germany—and making wigs from their blond hair, blond went from sinful to respectable.

1558, ENGLAND While Elizabeth was a natural redhead, hardly anyone else was (red is the rarest of hair colors). As the use of harsh dyes and bleaches, like lead and sulphuric acid, caused hairlines to recede, faces took on a heart shape—which became desirable. Hair dyes continued to burn and blister all the way until the early 1900s, when improved formulas were introduced by the French Harmless Hair Dye Company, later known as L'Oréal.

1624, FRANCE As wig styles developed after Louis XIII, white became the favorite color. The wealthy had their servants powder their wigs by blowing wheat flour with a bellows from the fireplace. With flour going every which way, the French invented a new room—a powder room (now called a bathroom) so they would have a place to powder without worrying about the mess. Today, mainly in England, lawyers and judges still wear these heavy white wigs.

1644, CHINA The switch to the Manchu ponytail, or queue, marked perhaps the fastest hairstyle change in history. Men who did not comply could be executed. In the 1870s, when Chinese men immigrated to California to work, some Americans made fun of the queues and even forcibly cut them off. Back in China, in 1912, the new revolutionary government deemed queues a symbol of the old ways and ordered all queues cut off—again, by force, if necessary.

ABOUT 1785, VERSAILLES, FRANCE Professional hairdressers were starting to replace barbers, and they were out of control. Having a towering French hairdo was like wearing a Christmas tree. Besides making an outstanding home for bugs, it could also catch on fire (several women died after brushing against chandeliers), cause tremendous headaches, and require doorways to be enlarged. Grooming it in public was acceptable—ladies would insert scratchers with long handles into it. As for Marie Antoinette, she lost her hair and her head in the French Revolution of 1789. Her hairdresser would have been executed along with her, but he managed to escape the country. To the poor and hungry, these insane hairdos were a symbol of the wealthy people they despised. And all that flour that powdered their hair—it could have been used for bread.

1789, UNITED STATES Washington used as much powder on his hair as one would use for a wig, and sometimes carelessly wore it on his shoulders as well. When fans requested locks of the great man's hair, he was rumored to comply by cutting the tails of his horses and giving away horsehair instead.

AROUND 1810, VIENNA, AUSTRIA Beethoven's hair became even more famous after his death. In 2000, chemical analysts found unusual amounts of lead in eight strands of his hair, and some believe lead poisoning may have caused his deafness and eventually his death.

1814, BRIGHTON, ENGLAND Before this, most people around the world did not wash their hair often (once a month at the very most) and when they did, the "shampoo" was sometimes urine or, more typically, lye—water mixed with ashes from the fireplace. Even as late as 1946, the *Encyclopædia Britannica* advised that hair needed washing only every other week.

1872, PARIS, FRANCE Ever since 1635, when the first hair salon for women opened in Paris, whatever happened in this high-fashion city set the trends in hair. For those unlucky enough to live outside it, dolls with the newest hairdos would be sent all over Europe.

1882, LOCKPORT, NEW YORK The Sutherland sisters had a total of 37 feet of hair among them. They probably did not use their father's "Hair Grower"—later, a chemical analysis showed that almost half of it was simply rum.

1905, DENVER, COLORADO One who got her start with Madam Walker was Marjorie Stewart Joyner of Chicago, who later invented a hair machine that made permanent waves. It was the birth of the perm, in 1928. Her machine had sixteen rods, normally used to cook pot roasts, now for cooking hair—for up to 12 hours, and only for the very rich. Joyner became the first African-American woman to be granted a patent.

AROUND 1906, UNITED STATES By 1920, there were hair-dryers in beauty shops—heavy, noisy machines that took more than an hour to do the job. The modern portable blow-dryer didn't arrive until 1971.

AROUND 1924, FRANCE A year later, Antoine opened the most famous salon in America, at Saks Fifth Avenue in New York City. One of his employees, Sydney Guilaroff, went on to Hollywood and became the first hairdresser for movie stars.

AROUND 1935, MEXICO Frida didn't mind having a unibrow—in fact, she used makeup to make it darker. Meanwhile, her husband, the famous artist Diego Rivera, was so careless with his hair that it often had splotches of paint in it.

1936, HOLLYWOOD, CALIFORNIA By now, more people were getting their hair ideas from what movie stars wore in Hollywood, not what the rich did in Paris. Fashions that used to last for centuries were now changing all the time.

1939, JAPAN A cure for baldness continues to baffle scientists. As of 2004, American men were spending over $1.3 *billion* a year trying to cope.

1961, DETROIT, MICHIGAN The following year, a high school girl in Canton, Ohio, left her beehive in place for weeks—until a classmate spotted a nest of cockroaches in it. This inspired many an urban legend combining spiders with hairdos. Still, by 1964, hairspray was the top-selling beauty product in America.

1964, LIVERPOOL, ENGLAND The 1960s were just huge for hair. One of the earliest Beatles fans, Astrid Kirchherr, persuaded them to ditch their greasy ducktails and adopt a moptop (actually a version of a typical upside-down bowl haircut from the early 1400s)—they found it very amusing at first. In 1967, a musical play all about hippies (and their long, flowing hair) premiered in New York—naturally, it was called *Hair*. In 1968, Jamaican singer Bob Marley started wearing his hair in dreadlocks that became trendy. By that year, wigs were a $500-million-a-year business in America, with Beatle moptop wigs some of the most popular. The famous American artist Andy Warhol was never seen without a moptop wig, and had a snap surgically implanted in his skull so he could snap his wigs on and off to suit his mood.

1974, GREENWICH, CONNECTICUT Hamill's wedge was actually a version of the five-point geometric cut, invented in 1964 at the London salon of the influential hairdresser Vidal Sassoon. His goal was to create neat, clean hairdos that were low maintenance compared to styles in the past.

1970S AND '80S, NEW YORK CITY AND LONDON When hair mousse was invented in 1983, it made punk hairstyles easier to manage.

2007, ENGLAND Hair care is now a major industry everywhere, and hairdressers have become celebrities. And in 2010 a new TV reality show began that starred "fantasy hair," an outrageous style popularized by singer Lady Gaga and others.

SOURCES

* Badt, Karin Luisa. *Hair There and Everywhere.* Chicago: Childrens Press, 1994.

Bryer, Robin. *The History of Hair: Fashion and Fantasy Down the Ages.* London: Philip Wilson Publishers, 2000.

+++ Corson, Richard. *Fashions in Hair: The First Five Thousand Years.* London: Peter Owen, 2001.

de Courtais, Georgine. *Women's Hats, Headdresses and Hairstyles, with 453 Illustrations, Medieval to Modern.* Mineola, NY: Dover, 1986.

* Lasky, Kathryn. *Vision of Beauty: The Story of Sarah Breedlove Walker.* New York: Candlewick, 2000.

* Lattimore, Deborah. *The Lady with the Ship on Her Head.* San Diego: Harcourt, 1990.

Sherrow, Victoria. *Encyclopedia of Hair: A Cultural History.* Westport, Conn.: Greenwood Press, 2006.

Simon, Diane. *Hair: Public, Political, Extremely Personal.* New York: St. Martin's, 2000.

* Swain, Ruth Freeman. *Hairdo! What We Do and Did to Our Hair.* New York: Holiday House, 2002.

Weitz, Rose. *Rapunzel's Daughters: What Women's Hair Tells Us About Women's Lives.* New York: Farrar, Straus and Giroux, 2004.

* especially for young readers

+++ best book for picture research